I0626893

There is no other book that introduces kids to the ancient art of Tai Chi in a way that is fun, accessible, and perfectly tailored to their age and energy. Tai Chi for Kids helps kids discover the joy of movement and mindfulness. And it works! With clear instructions, playful illustrations, and imaginative exercises, this book empowers kids to explore balance, focus, and relaxation while having a great time. Cari has also included audio guided movements for kids to use on their own. Tai Chi for Kids is more than a book—it's a journey into health, confidence, and a lifelong love of mindful movement. As a child and family therapist for thirty years, I have yet to find a more creative and timely book to help kids manage the unparalleled stress they experience in these times.

—Kathy Hegberg, M.A.,
Child and Family Therapist,
Founder of Focused Kids

This is one of the most valuable resources any parent or teacher could have in their backpack. Tai Chi for Kids is an interactive playground of spontaneous fun, laughter, and all-around healthy activity for kids of all ages, tried and tested for decades across the globe by this wise educator. But wait! Please don't think for one second that this is just another exercise book to slide onto your shelf or get buried in a pile on your desk! Your phone unlocks the secret sauce that offers you and your kids a gift. Who knew movement could be so much fun? After years of playing with kids impacted by disasters in countries all over the world, I know that this is one of the most valuable resources any parent, teacher, or relief worker could have in their backpack.

—William Spear, Founder,
Second Response for Treatment of Trauma

In times of record stress for our kids, what they need is more movement and mindfulness. An experienced and established educator with decades of experience, Cari Shurman's guide to Tai Chi is just what today's youth need. A clear, skillful guide to learning the basic principles of Tai Chi.

—Dr. Christopher Willard,
Lecturer in Psychiatry, Harvard Medical School

Tai Chi's profound health benefits have dramatically increased its popularity among older adults in the West. However, its potential benefits for children have been greatly under-appreciated. Leveraging her many years as a dedicated educator and student of Tai Chi, Cari Shurman's book, Tai Chi for Kids, *is a playful and practical tool for teachers and parents wanting to apply Tai Chi's wisdom to enhance the resilience, curiosity, and health of our children facing an increasingly stressful and challenging world.*

—Peter Wayne, Ph.D., author
The Harvard Medical School Guide to Tai Chi

Cari's Tai Chi classes are always popular here at Rancho La Puerta. They are user friendly, and very calming. Our youth are overwhelmed with stress that we did not experience at their ages. Tai Chi is a perfect tool they can learn early and continue through life. Learning to control our inner environment is life enhancing.

—Barry Shingle, Director,
Rancho La Puerta

Bravo Cari! The best investment we can make in the world today is in our children. Being a Senior Qigong teacher for over 30 years, I so honor your focus on the young angels who will inherit our world, supporting their caring parents in the process.

—Francesco Garri Garripoli,
author of The Qi Effect, and founder of CommunityAwake

Cari Shurman is the best person to write this book. Her vast experience in teaching Tai Chi to kids of all ages started in 1995 at our wellness center in Miami, Florida. As a physician, I saw how Tai Chi helped children feel happier. From age three, many are addicted to cell phones and social media. This increases depression and anxiety. With the guidance of this book, caregivers and kids can do Tai Chi daily and see a happier, more focused child with improved health and quality of life.

—Nilza Kallos, MD,
Women's Breast Health Center, Miami

Tai Chi for Kids

AND THE ADULTS WHO LOVE THEM

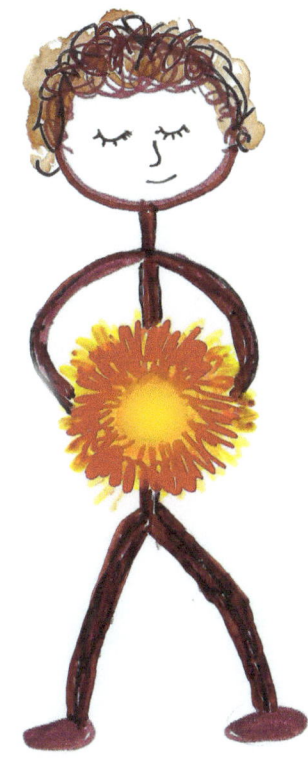

Written and Illustrated
by Cari Shurman

Tai Chi for Kids © 2025 by Cari Shurman

Written and Illustrated by Cari Shurman

All rights reserved. No part of this book may be reproduced by any mechanical, photographic, or electronic process, or in the form of a phonographic recording; nor may it be stored in a retrieval system, transmitted, or otherwise be copied for public or private use —other than for "fair use" as brief quotations embodied in articles and reviews— without prior written permission of the author/publisher.

Published by Tai Chi for Kids, Inc.
Carbondale, Colorado

Paperback ISBN: 979-8-9985876-0-3
Hardcover ISBN: 979-8-9985876-2-7
eBook ISBN: 979-8-9985876-1-0

Library of Congress Control Number: 2025907261

Light of the Moon, Inc.
Empowering Independent Authors Since 2009
Book Design/Production/Consulting
Glenwood Springs, Colorado
www.lightofthemooninc.com

To the thousands of kids
who have done Tai Chi for Kids with me.
I always love seeing your expressions relax as we
share the calmness and peace of Tai Chi.

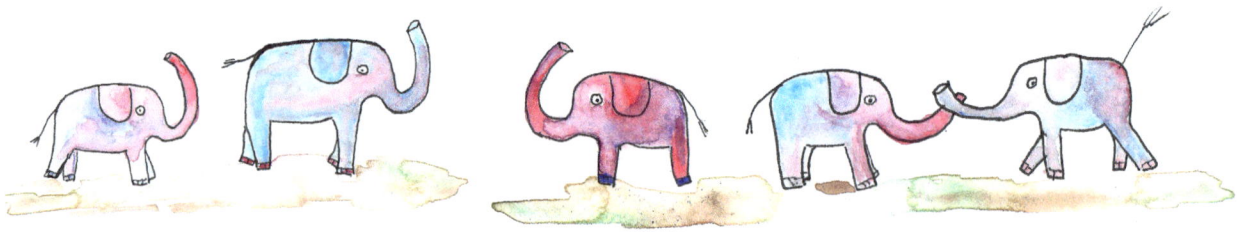

To all who love and care for kids,

Open up this book with your kids when it seems like it's time for a break from the stress of daily life. We all need breaks from our phones, obligations, and the unforgiving fast pace of life. We need a quiet, peaceful time every day to get the most out of whatever we are doing.

We need to connect to our *chi*—the energy in our body. When we feel our *chi* flowing, we are calm and focused. The breathing, visualization, and movements of Tai Chi help us find those quiet moments.

In my 25 years of teaching Tai Chi for Kids© I have observed that children of all ages are able to:

- Slow down and breathe
- Focus and learn
- Develop self-confidence
- Feel peaceful and happy

I hope you enjoy the moves I suggest here. I do some of these moves every day. Please let me know if you have questions. I would love to hear from you.

Best wishes,
Cari Shurman
taichiforkids@gmail.com
www.taichiforkids.com

Why Tai Chi for Kids? Why Now?

There are so many reasons, starting with:
- There's way too much anxiety and depression in kids' lives.
- Kids often feel unfocused, anxious, nervous, or scared.
- Many kids struggle to get a good night's sleep.

Multiple studies from organizations including the World Health Organization and NCCIH/National Institute of Health, show that Tai Chi can help solve these issues in a healthy way. Check my website for details of these studies: www.taichiforkids.com/medical-studies-tai-chi

Tai Chi for Kids is easy to learn and fun to do. It can be just what we need in these challenging times. I have adapted traditional Tai Chi forms so that kids can easily relate to them. The poems and illustrations are suggestions of the moves. The audio-guide makes it even easier. As kids begin to focus and move, they feel the *chi* flowing in their bodies—in their hands, feet, and tummies. The calmness allows their imagination to grow. Kids "become" the elephant in Africa and the crane flying over the wetlands.

Moving as animals allows kids to relax and let go of expectations. Tai Chi takes them to a different place with **no competition and no demanding requirements.** The relaxed imagery is happy. Kids feel self-confident.

I think you will find *Tai Chi for Kids* rewarding for you and your child. Tai Chi is for everyone and any age.

How To Use and Enjoy *Tai Chi for Kids*

Each chapter in this book teaches a different Tai Chi move. There is a poem accompanying each move, a simple drawing to suggest the action, and an audio to guide the movement. (You can access the audio with the QR code.)

- Start by reading the poem and talking about it. What does it convey? What is *chi?* Are there different kinds of energy? Try moving as you hear the poem.
- Use the QR code for each move to listen to the audio guide. At times, you might close your eyes to really feel the movement.
- Ask some questions.
  — What did you feel?
  — Where did you feel your energy, your *chi*?
  — Could you see the color of the energy?

You may be surprised by the answers. Try another move.
You can do them in any order, at any time.
Every move should feel good. We aren't trying to do things faster or harder.
We want to be gentle, relaxed, strong, and focused.

It is best not to make corrections or suggestions. We all have our own interpretation. Children have particularly vivid imaginations. **Let the imagination and the chi guide you.** There is a special feeling inside when we trust and follow our own imagination.

Because this book is for a variety of ages, there might be a few words that younger children aren't familiar with. Please tell them that the abdomen is the tummy. Inhale and exhale mean breathe in and out. And visualize means imagine. They will catch on very quickly and be able to use those words themselves.

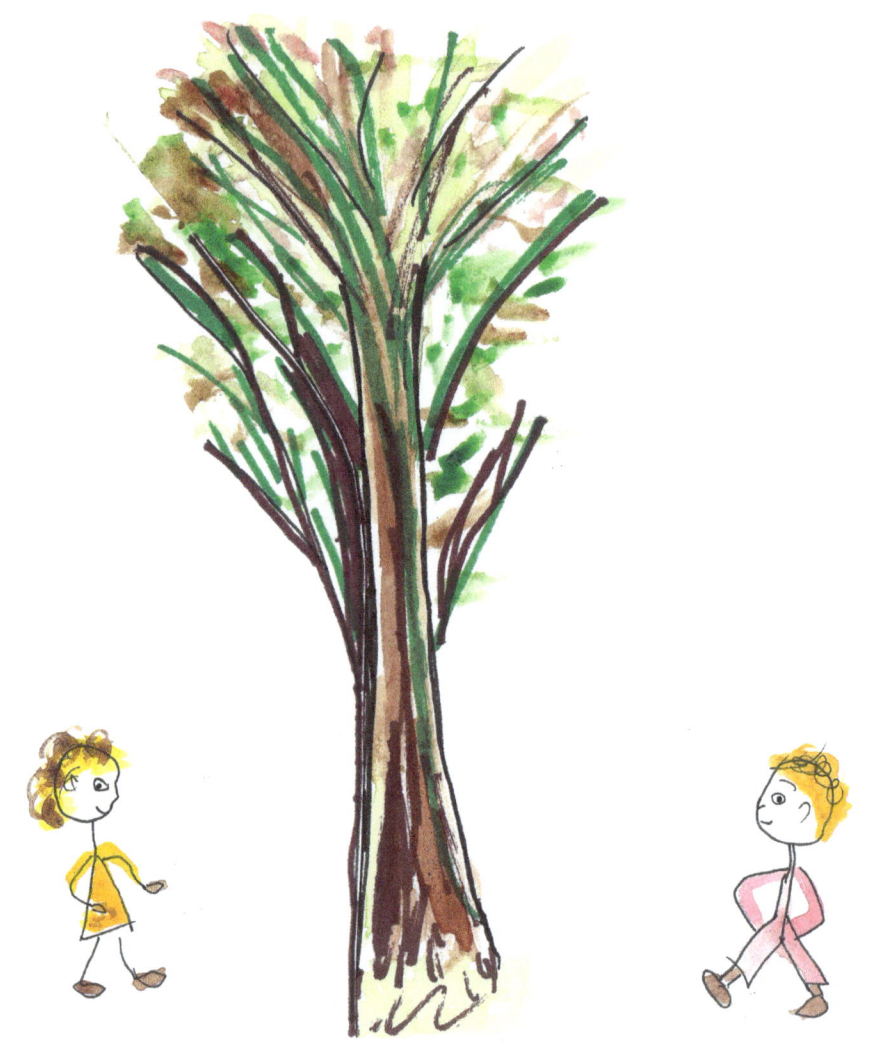

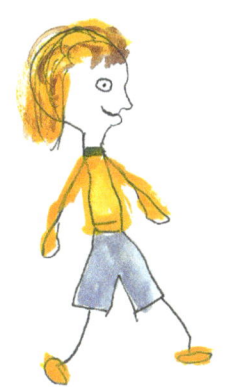

Let's Do
Tai Chi

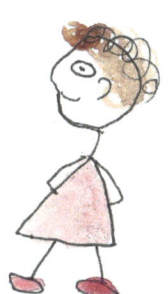

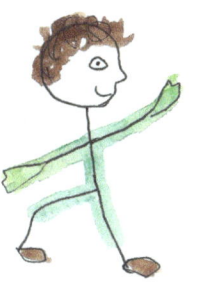

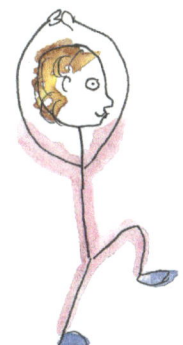

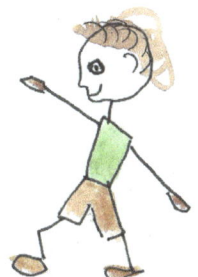

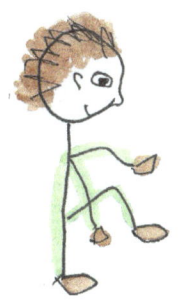

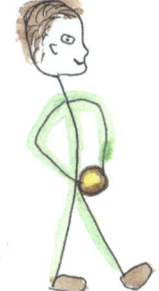

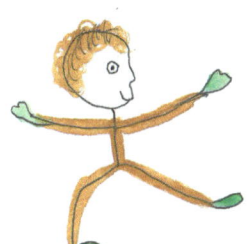

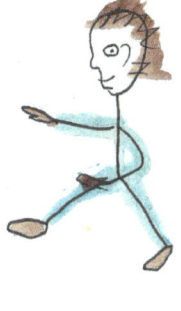

1. Waking Up Your Energy

In the morning, when I'm tired,
I can't feel my energy.
I tap here and there to wake it up.
It is my very own personal *chi*.

I tap all over my body,
my arms, my legs, my tummy.
Chi moves from my head to my toes.
It makes me feel happy and sunny.

Then I shake my tummy and feet.
It's really fun, you'll see!
Can you tap and shake your body,
to be focused and ready like me?

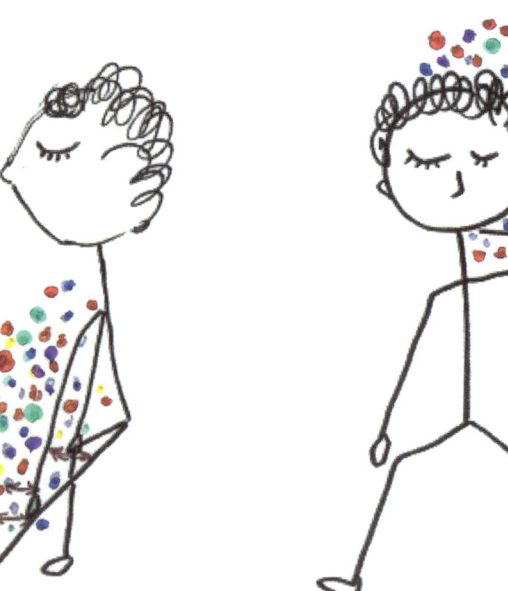

After shaking, I feel the *chi*,
in my toes, my legs, and my chest.
It keeps moving, it doesn't stop.
But when I'm *still*, it feels the best.

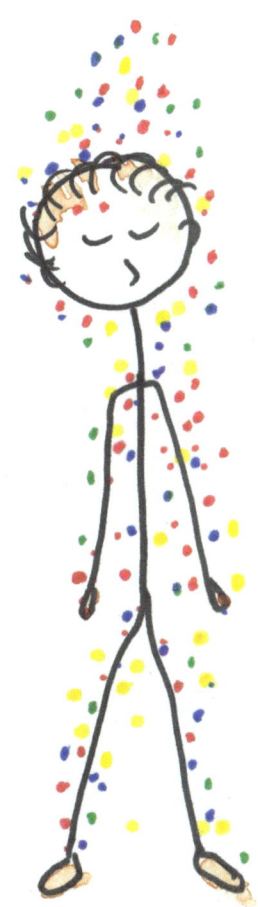

Waking Up
Your Energy
– Audio Guide

2. The Elephant Drinks Water

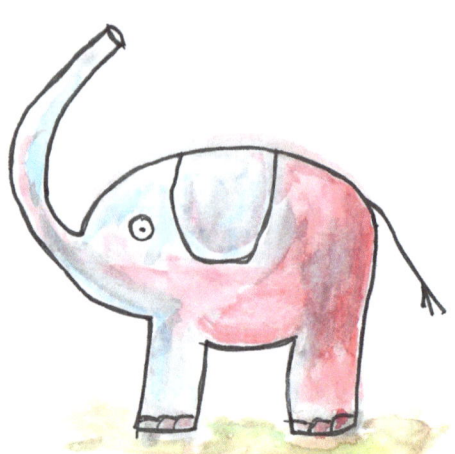

I am a little elephant in Africa,
growing up big and strong.
I walk with my family to the watering hole.
My trunk is soooo very long.

I stretch my trunk up high.
I love to sniff the air.
I suck water from the pond,
and spray it here and there.

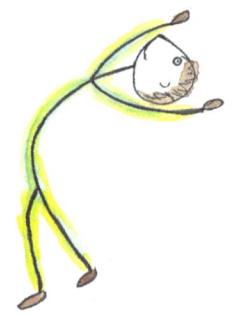

The water is so nice and cool.
I rest lying under a tree.
Can you be an African elephant, too?
An elephant just like me?

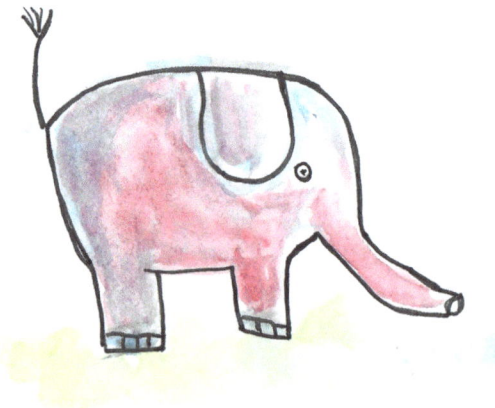

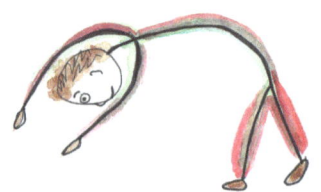

I bring the water up to my tummy.
I connect to the earth's strong *chi*.
Then up to my heart and my head.
I love the warm energy.

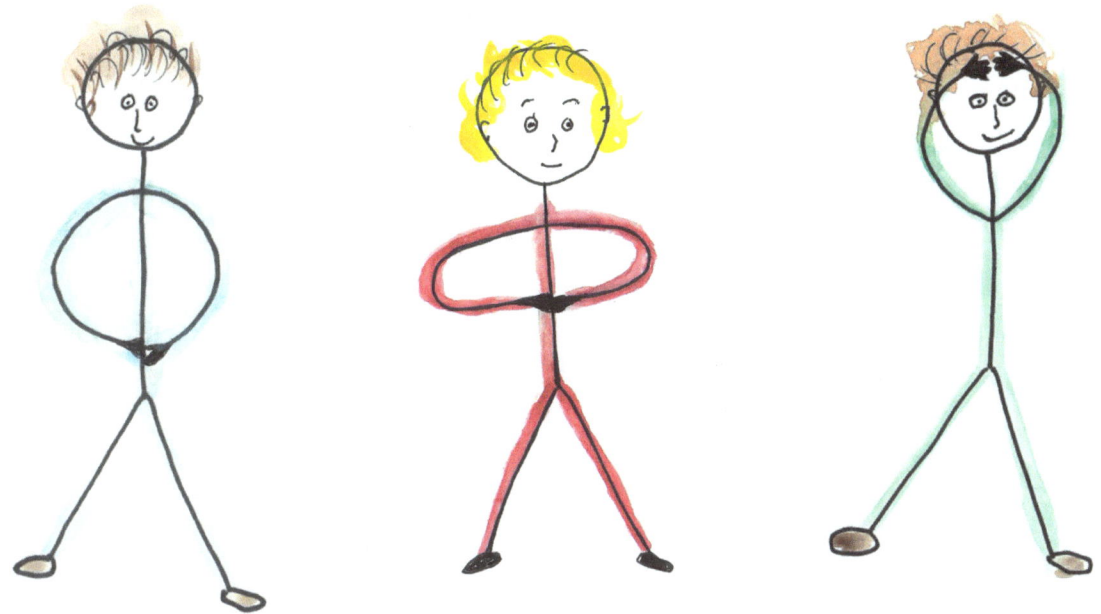

The Elephant
Drinks Water
– Audio Guide

3. Shooting a Bow and Arrow

I want to be like the archer,
who can shoot an arrow far.
Who is strong and very powerful,
and can focus on a star.

I pull the bow string back.
I focus with my eye.
I watch with my imagination.
I can see the arrow fly.

Let's shoot the arrow together,
with the target in our view.
Hold your breath, bend your knees.
I know you can focus, too.

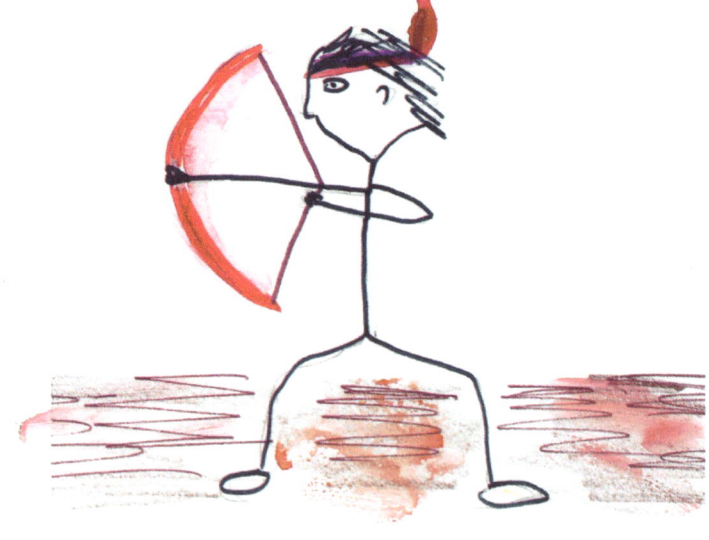

I bend and straighten my finger,
nine times to move the energy.
Now my tummy feels much better,
relaxed, and full of *chi*.

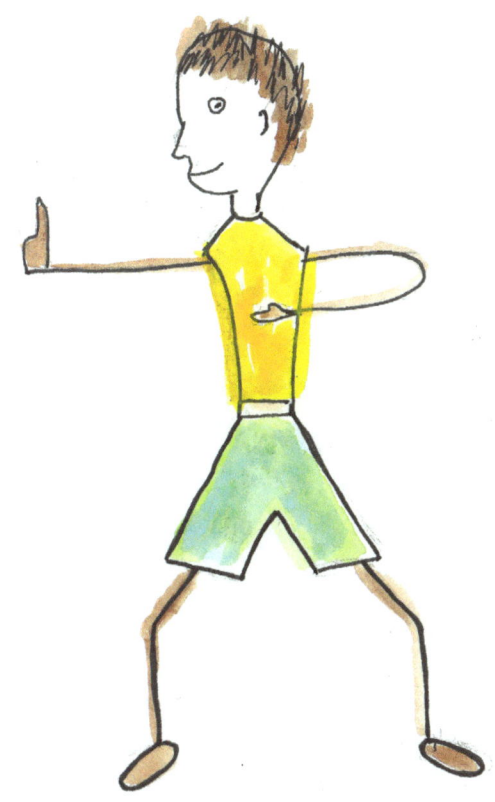

The Bow
and Arrow
– Audio Guide

4. Birds' Beaks

I put my fingers and thumb together,
to make beaks. Can you see?
The birds fly around me in circles,
and one sits right behind me.

The other one flies to the ground,
circling around my feet,
pecking at leaves and grass,
looking for something to eat.

Stretching the *chi* up slowly,
standing on my toes,
then flying down to the earth,
there is *chi* from my feet to my nose.

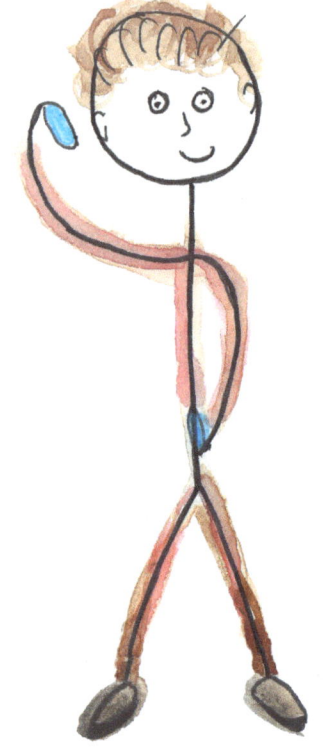

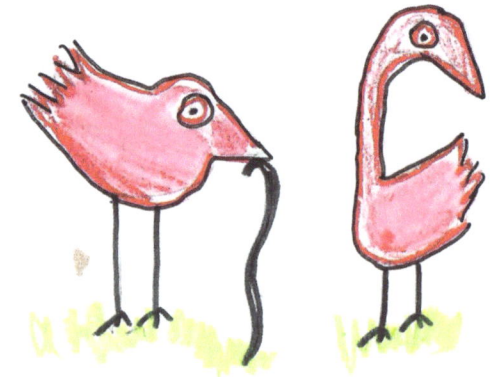

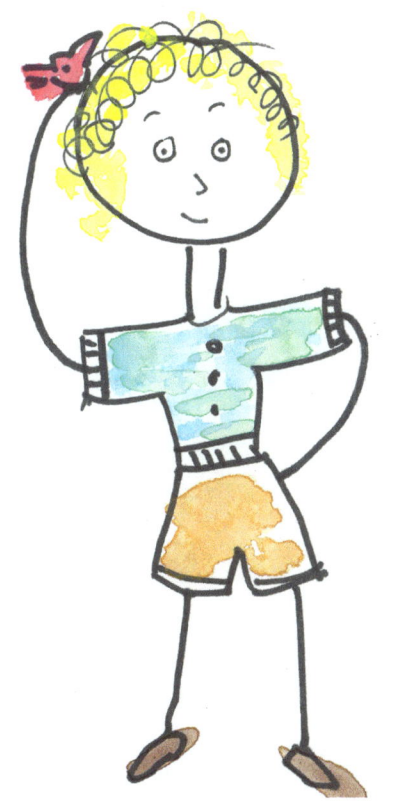

One bird sits on my back.
The other flies up to the sky.
I stand up tall on my toes.
I think that I, too, want to fly.

The Birds' Beaks
– Audio Guide

5. Embrace a Tree

The tree is so very tall.
It reaches way up to the sky.
I put my arms around the trunk.
It is strong and oh so high.

I feel my roots grow deep,
far down into the ground.
I gently sway in the breeze,
and the wind softly blows all around.

I'm a tree alone in the woods,
so tall and straight and calm.
I stretch my arms like branches,
and feel the *chi* of the tree in my palm.

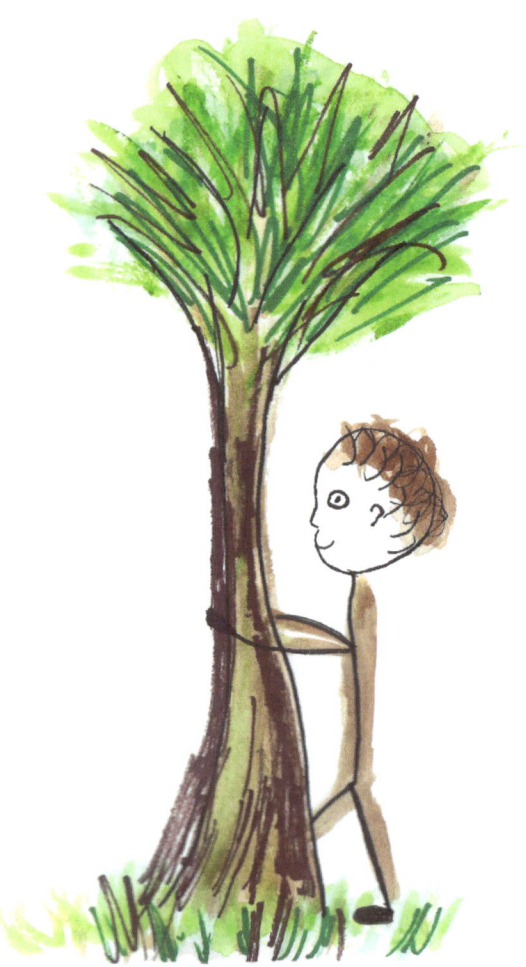

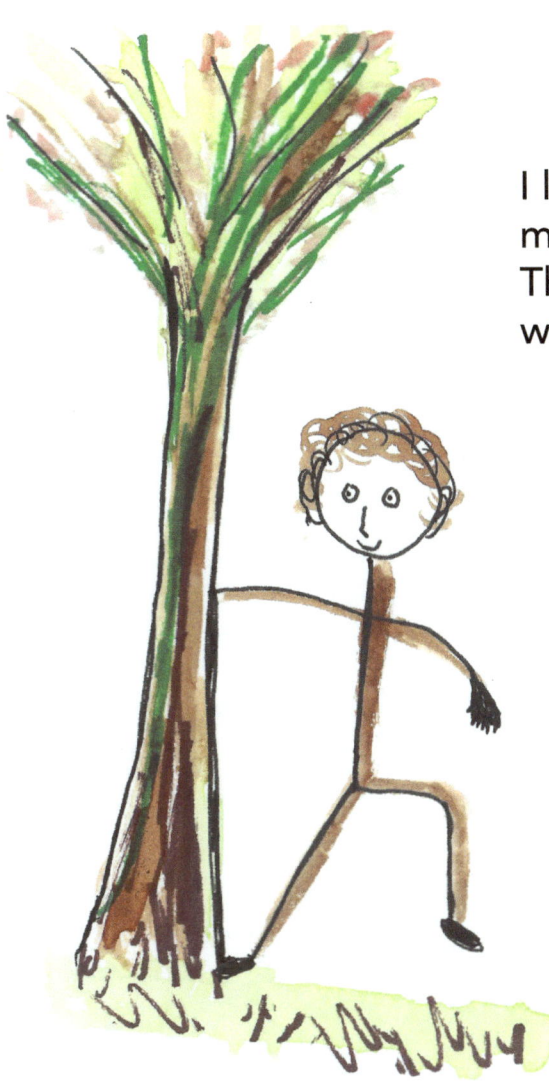

I lift my foot to stretch the roots,
my branches and leaves blowing free.
Then I balance and lift the other foot,
with the *chi* of the tree inside me.

Embrace
a Tree
– Audio Guide

6. The Crane Stands on One Leg and Flies

From the mountain I look around
at the hills so far below.
I see houses, trees and lakes,
and rivers that gently flow.

I feel the breeze under my wings.
Bending forward, I start to fly.
I lift one leg to the back.
I love flying up so high.

I soar down to the town below,
passing trees and birds as I fly.
I do it again on the other leg,
from the top of the mountain so high.

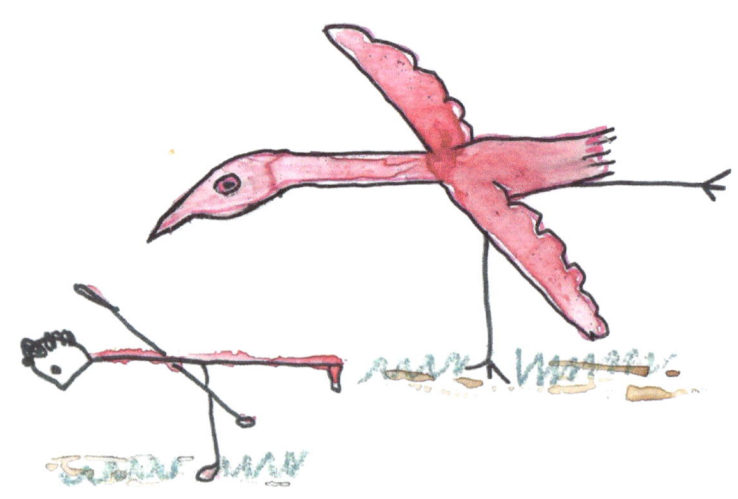

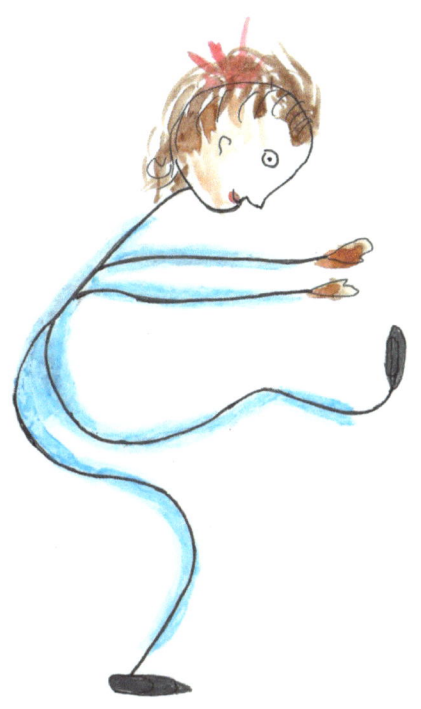

Then I stretch my leg to the front.
I am balanced and strong and light.
My energy flows all around.
I have had a beautiful flight.

The Crane Stands
on One Leg and Flies
– Audio Guide

7. The Lion Sleeps

Sometimes lions are sleepy.
Sometimes I'm tired, too.
I put my head down on my knee,
and lie there with nothing to do!

Then I yawn and look around.
I see the birds in the sky.
They fly up above my head.
I lie down and close my eyes.

I open my eyes and stretch.
Looking up, what do I see?
I see the clouds and the birds,
and lie back down on my knee.

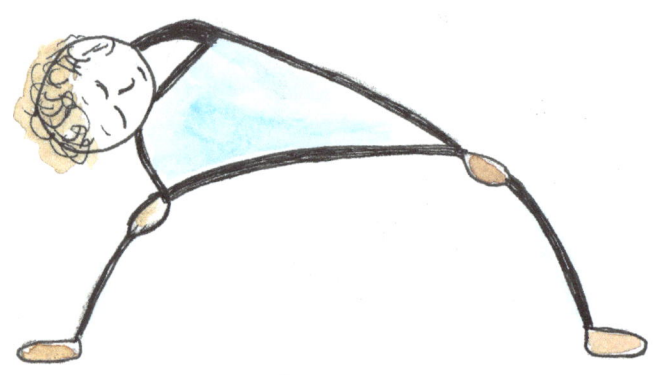

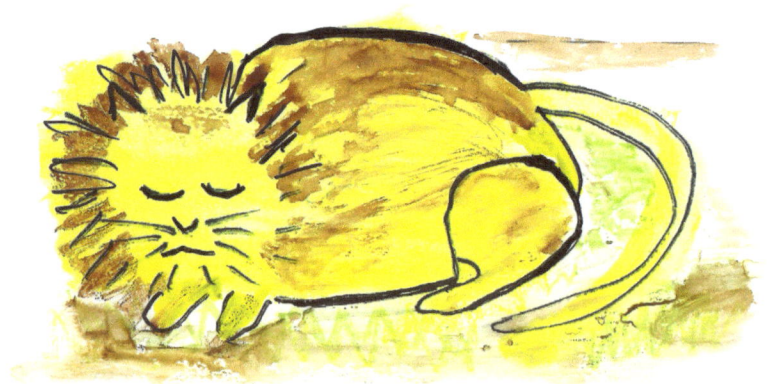

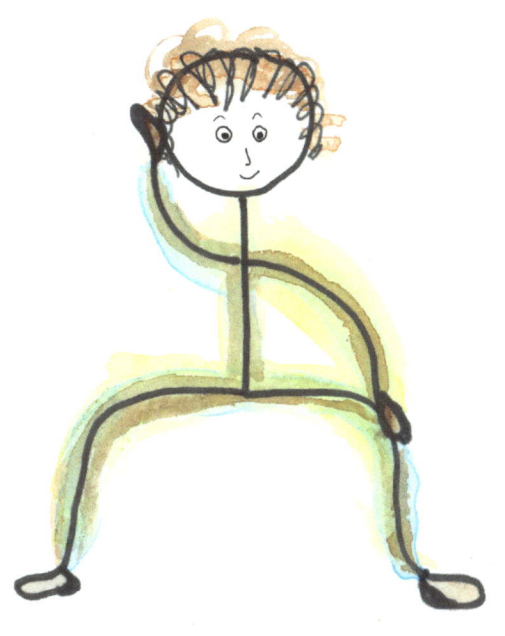

I open my mouth with a yawn.
No noise, not even a peep.
I make a pillow with my hand,
and fall right back asleep.

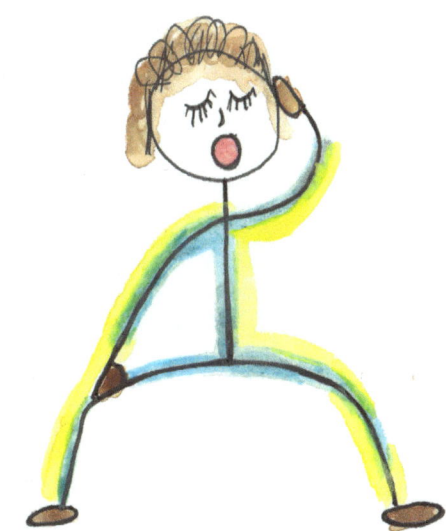

The Lion Sleeps
– Audio Guide

8. The Energy Ball

I reach my arms up high,
to find a ball of *chi*.
I bring it down to my chest.
It's like floating in an energy sea.

I close my eyes to see the ball.
I feel it soft and warm.
The color changes sometimes.
I roll it and feel the form.

I love to sleep with a chi ball,
in my heart, my head, or my tummy.
It makes me feel warm and nice,
and soft and peaceful and sunny.

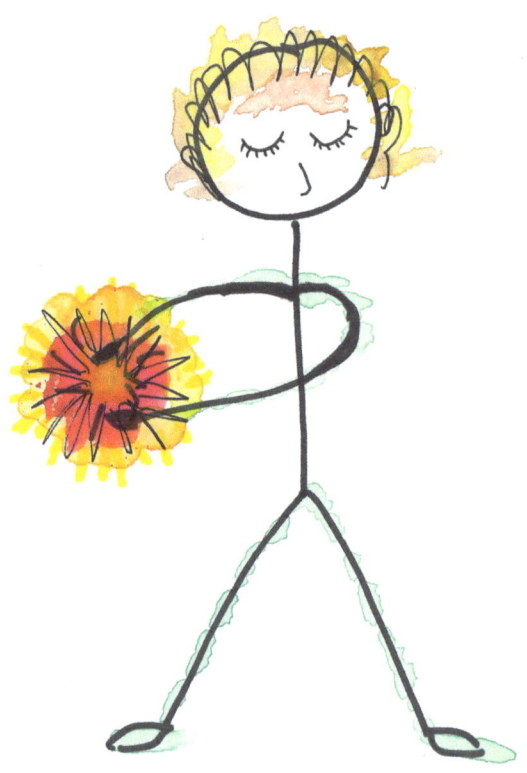

I put the energy deep inside,
in my heart and in my head.
I make an energy ball every night
and sleep with it in my bed.

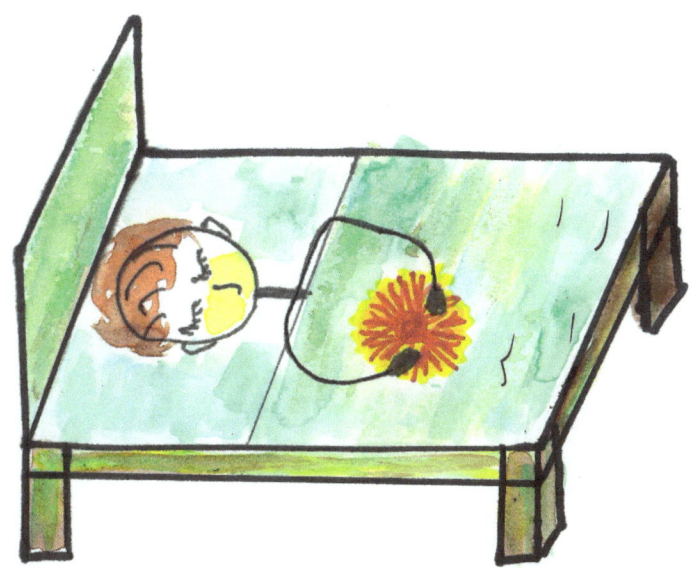

The Energy Ball
– Audio Guide

Why Does Tai Chi Work So Well?

These moves come from thousands of years of observation and study in China of how animals move, how the *chi*—the energy—flows in nature and in our body. This is the basis of Traditional Chinese Medicine. It became evident that through breathing, visualization, and movement we can improve the flow of *chi*. This helps us to be strong and healthy, to focus better, and to feel happy. Each move works on a different part of the body, but they all work together for better health.

Kids love to focus and sleep like a lion. They actually feel rested after the lion takes a nap. Focusing your mind makes the *chi* feel more powerful and helps with relaxation.

I suggest that you do not correct the child during the moves. In many cases, the child may have a different image from yours. And it may change from time to time. **The most important part of the move is the focus of the mind and the imagery.**

What Happens in My Body When I Do Tai Chi?

Each move is based on the energy flow along the meridians of the body to all our cells. The movements help us relax, which in turn increases the energy flow.

1. Waking up My Energy

Sometimes our *chi* is stuck or tired. It helps if we wake it up in the morning. By tapping on the body and shaking all over, we send *chi* to all the muscles, organs, bones, nerves, etc. We are ready for the activities of the day. We can do this at various times during the day to shake out tension, stiffness, and even frustration.

2. The Elephant Drinks Water

This move helps build a flexible, strong spine. The elephant bends forward and arches back—but not too much—just enough to feel good. We feel the water energy rising to our three energy centers: the belly—just below the navel, the heart center —in the middle of the chest, and the third eye—between our eyebrows. The energy gives us strength and stability, and a strong connection to the earth.

3. The Bow and Arrow

We root our feet with a relaxed but straight spine. We are strong as we pull the bow string back. Our lungs expand taking in extra oxygen and energy. Our focus is on the target: our index finger pointing up. Focusing on the target helps us focus on other activities during the day. Bending and straightening the index finger is good for our digestive system.

4. Birds' Beaks

We move with graceful coordination. Our balance improves as we rise onto our toes. Connecting to the *yin* energy of the earth through our roots gives us calmness, coolness, and stability. Stretching up, we connect to the bright, warm, active *yang* energy of the heavens. We look for the balance of the *yin* and the *yang*, the slow and the fast, the warm and the cool, in everything we do. We move the energy through our body for balance.

5. Embrace a Tree

With roots growing from our feet into the earth, we can be as centered and peaceful as a tree. Trees are strong and calm. The connection to the earth through the roots gives security and peace. Balance improves as we slowly lift our foot, stretching the root. When we focus on our roots we energize the kidneys. We feel powerful and tall like a tree.

6. The Crane Stands on One Leg and Flies

This move involves balance, focus, and strength. We root our feet and focus on those roots. Focusing our eyes on a point on the ground gives even better balance. As we soar down over the valley we relax. Our imagination makes it feel like we are really flying. Lifting your leg to the back and then moving it to the front improves balance and muscle control. Physical and emotional balance are closely connected.

7. The Lion Sleeps

Lying down on one knee improves the circulation in our whole body, from our legs to our torso and to our head. Then we lie down on the other knee. We are improving inner harmony, flexibility, and recovery from activities. The focused breathing relaxes our body and energizes the organs. It is a peaceful break in our day.

8. The Energy Ball

We feel rooted, strong, secure, peaceful, and connected to the earth and the nature around us. The color of the energy ball may change. It may be a different color on different days. We can stand inside the energy ball. It feels safe and peaceful in this beautiful space. It allows us to focus and relax different parts of our body as we feel the energy move through and around us. It can help us fall asleep. The warm energy helps develop self-confidence.

Going Deeper with *Tai Chi for Kids*

Below you'll find two additional QR codes. One is labeled "Morning Session" and includes the audio guides for moves one through four. The other is labeled "Evening Session" and includes the audio guides for moves five through eight. You can choose one of these for a longer session. In the morning, ten minutes of Tai Chi is the perfect way to get ready for the day. School is better when your *chi* is flowing. After school you can relax with whichever moves you like best. And at night, as part of your nighttime routine, do moves five through eight. You can start by doing the movements standing up. Then repeat the audio while lying in bed, visualizing the moves. It becomes a meditation, which prepares you for sleep. Establishing a routine like this is a powerful way to end the day.

Morning Session,
11 minutes,
Audio Guides #1-4

Evening Session,
11 minutes,
Audio Guides #5-8

The following pages show the scripts of the eight different Audio Guides. These can be used to make your own recording, if you wish.

#1 WAKING UP YOUR ENERGY audio script

Stand with your feet shoulder width apart. Using your hands to tap on your legs, go up the inside and down the outside of each leg. Tap on the top of your foot. Come up your legs again; all the way up and all the way down. Every time you tap you are helping the energy move better through your body. And you are helping any pain move away, out of your body. Be very quiet. Listen to the sound of your tapping. Tap on your groin where your legs join your body and on your abdomen. Can you feel the energy moving in your legs and in your tummy?

Tap under one arm down the side of your body, up to the middle of your chest and around again. Now go down your arm to your hand and up the back of your arm to your shoulder. Down your arm to your hand and up the back of your arm to your shoulder. And let's go to the other side. Under your arm tapping, tapping, tapping down to your waist, around, and tap on your chest. Under your arm, down and around and tap on your chest.

Tap on your arm all the way down to your palm and up the back to your shoulder.

Tap hard on your shoulder to break up any tension. Now close your eyes and with one hand at the back of your neck, tap just at your hairline like a woodpecker tapping a hole in a tree.

Keep your eyes closed. Feel your body relax and let all the tightness melt away. Now use your other hand to tap on your neck. Be sure your jaw is very loose, and all the muscles of your face are soft. Now reach behind your back and tap on either side of your spine. Be careful not to hit your spine, but just tap either side, up and down over your kidneys. Can you feel the warm energy under your hands? Every time you tap on your body, you help the energy move all over your body.

Let's wake up our ears. Pull and stretch and squeeze your ears. Run your fingers all around the curves and folds of your ears. Pull and stretch in all directions. Feel the energy surge through your whole body.

Now shake. Shake very hard to get rid of any bad energy. Shake and shake and shake. Let it move out. Let it go out your feet, out your fingers. All the stiffness melts away. Begin to tap lightly on your head with your fingers like raindrops falling on your head. Close your eyes. Let the rain drip down your face, your shoulders, your chest, your tummy, your back. You're washing in a beautiful light rain shower. It leaves you sparkling clean. Stand in the sun to dry off.

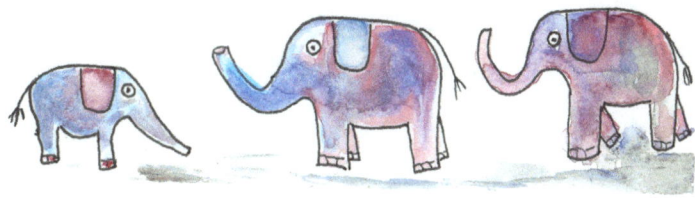

#2 The Elephant Drinks Water audio script

Elephants are big, heavy, magnificent animals with very long trunks. Make a trunk with your arms and reach way out in front of you, rounding your back, and dropping your head. Now turn your palms up and pull your arms back by your waist, behind your back. Arch and look up. Stretch forward, reaching your arms out like an elephant's trunk, smelling everything around you.

Pull the trunk back. Bring your hands behind you, arching your back. Touch your fingers together behind your back. Stretch your trunk forward. Inhale. Exhale as you pull your arms back. Arch. Look up. Breathe in the energy and feel it pass through your whole body.

And now we've come to the watering hole. Let your trunk hang down, very long and loose, just above the ground. Let it swing a little side to side. It's such a hot sunny day. We're very thirsty.

With our trunks, we drink some water. Sucking in the water, breathe in and slowly pull it up to your tummy. Lower your trunk, breathe out, and get more water. Breathe in as you bring the water up to your chest. Breathe out as you slowly drop your trunk back down to the water.

Once more, suck the water all the way up in your trunk, moving your trunk to your forehead. Then lower your trunk again. One last time, bring the water up to the top of your head. Pour it over your whole body with your trunk, showering in the wonderful cool water. How clean you feel.

Shake off your body to dry and stand for a moment in the sun.

#3 Shooting A Bow and Arrow audio script

Stand with your feet shoulder width apart. Your index finger pointing up will be your target.

As you inhale, reach forward with rounded arms to gather the energy into a big ball. Pull it toward your chest. As you exhale, bend both knees and extend your right arm out to the side. Pull the bowstring back with your left arm. Focus all of your attention on the index finger of your right hand pointing up. Hold the position. Release the bow string and relax.

Stand straight. Gather the energy again as you inhale. Pull it into your chest. Extend your left arm straight out to the side. Pull the bowstring back with your right arm. Feel your chest open. Bend both knees. Be sure your spine is straight. Hold the position. Focus on your index finger pointing up. Release the bowstring as you shoot the arrow. Relax and stand straight.

Once again, gather the energy. Pull it into your chest. Extend your right arm. Your weight is evenly distributed over both feet. Your knees are bent. Focus on the target. Open your chest. Hold the position. Stare at your finger. Release the bow string.

Stand straight. Gather the energy again into your chest. Bend both knees, extend your left arm to the side. Focus your attention on your target. Feel the weight evenly distributed between your feet. Feel the strength in your arms and your legs. Feel your connection to the earth. Release the bowstring and stand straight again.

Once more shoot to the right. Gather the energy. Extend your right arm. Bend your knees. Hold the position. While you focus on your index finger, bend and straighten it nine times. Feel the energy surge through your body. Release the bowstring.

Stand straight. Gather the energy again. Pull it into your chest. Extend your arm to the left. Bend your knees. Hold the position. Focus on your index finger. Now bend and straighten your finger nine times. Release. Stand up straight. Drop your arms to your side. Shake your legs to relax.

#4 The Birds' Beaks audio script

Make birds' beaks with your wrists. Put all the fingers and thumb of one hand together and bend your wrist down. Do the same thing with the other wrist. Move your left hand behind you. The bird flies around to sit on your back with the beak pointed up. Using the bird's beak of your right hand, let the bird circle around and around going down to the earth. The strong beak twists through the threads of energy growing from the earth.

Grabbing the energy, the bird slowly rises, pulling the energy up to your chest with a long slow inhalation. Feel the energy rise in your body. Pull it up to your forehead. Rise carefully onto your toes. Hold your balance for a moment. Focus on the contact of your feet with the earth so you don't fall. Slowly come down and let the bird's beak go back to the earth with a long slow exhalation.

Stand straight and change hands. Move your right hand behind you to let the bird sit on your back. Bend forward and drop the bird's beak of your left hand down to the earth. The beak twists around and around the threads of energy growing from the earth.

The bird grabs the energy from the earth and begins to stretch it up the front of your body. With a long slow inhalation stretch the energy all the way up to your forehead. Lift carefully onto your toes. Hold for a moment and slowly lower the bird's beak back to the earth as you exhale.

Stand straight. Begin to turn from the waist and let one bird stretch his long neck up and behind you over your shoulder, his beak pointing down. He stretches to look at the moon. Exhale and the bird returns to your chest.

Now the other bird stretches his long neck up, beak pointing down. He turns to the back. Look over your shoulder, twisting from the waist, looking at the moon, and the bird returns to your chest. Lower your arms to your sides, close your eyes and focus on the breath. Relax your shoulders. Let your hands hang loose. Feel the beauty of nature around you. Be aware of the energy circulating around and through your body.

#5 Embrace a Tree audio script

Stand tall and straight, but without forcing your body. Feel like a tree. Close your eyes and feel roots growing from the bottoms of your feet into the earth. Let the roots grow from the little depression near the middle of your foot, just behind the ball of your foot. That point is called the *Bubbling Well*. Visualize the roots growing into the ground, deeper and deeper. Keep your eyes closed. Try to notice how deep the roots can go.

You might begin to feel the energy from the earth coming into your foot just as a tree absorbs nutrients from the earth. Raise your arms straight out in front of you softly rounded as if you were holding them around a tree trunk. Stand for a moment breathing calmly.

Feel the energy going around and around your arms. Begin to absorb the energy from the trunk of the tree. Relax your shoulders. Relax your jaw. Let your arms float up like the branches of a tree. Feel leaves begin to grow from the branches. Relax your arms and let them come slowly back to your sides.

Focus on your roots again. Feel the tree sway slightly in the breeze.

Now, lift one foot a few inches off the ground, stretching the root and then let the root pull your foot back to the earth. Lift the other foot a little bit, stretching the root and return it to the earth. Lift each foot again, stretching the roots. The roots keep you balanced and stable.

Stand tall and straight. Slowly let your arms reach up, softly rounded like the branches of the tree. Lower them to your sides. Relax.

#6 The Crane Stands on One Leg and Flies audio script

Stand with your feet shoulder width apart. Let your knees soften. Your feet are parallel. Your spine is long and straight. Slowly lift your arms like wings, letting them float up above your shoulders. As they slowly float down, feel the breeze through your fingers.

Once more raise your wings and lower them to your sides. Visualize the roots growing from the bottoms of your feet into the earth. Notice how deep they go, what they look like, how they feel.

Now place all of your weight on your right foot. Bend your knee very slightly, just so it isn't tight. Your eyes are open, staring at a spot on the ground. As you inhale, begin to lift your left leg. Stretch it behind you. Lean forward. Exhale. Spread your wings. Stretch your left leg a little higher. Your balance will be stronger if you keep all of your attention on your roots and your eyes focused on a spot on the earth. Feel yourself flying. Now slowly come up and extend your left leg to the front. Reach your hands out in front of you, toward your foot. Hold for a moment. Flap your wings and slowly lower your left leg to the earth.

Stand tall and straight, with all of your weight on your left foot. Take a moment to focus on the root. Feel it grow into the earth. Your eyes are open, staring at the ground. Slowly lift your right leg. Spread your wings. As you exhale, stretch your right leg behind you, bending forward. Hold the position. Keep your eyes focused on the floor. Keep the picture of your roots clear in your mind. You are flying.

Slowly come up and extend your right leg in front of you. Reach your hands toward your extended leg. Flap your wings once and slowly lower your leg to the earth. Stand straight and tall. Lift your wings one more time. Lower your arms to your sides. Feel how long and straight your spine is. Feel how you are rooted to the earth.

#7. The Lion Sleeps audio script

Sometimes lions feel very lazy. Let's open our legs very wide and sleep like a lion.

Bend both of your knees sinking down. Place the backs of your hands on your knees. The lion falls asleep on one side. Rest your head on one of your bent knees. Then, yawning and stretching, the lion comes up and falls asleep on the other side. The lion stretches up once more, inhaling as he makes a big yawn and falls asleep to the first side. Relax and breathe.

One more time he changes his position coming up. Yawning, he lies down. Exhale and fall asleep.

Lions like it if you make a pillow for them. They sleep even better.

Place the back of one hand against your cheek. As you exhale, lie down on your knee using your hand as a pillow. Close your eyes and rest. The lion sleeps a bit and then he opens his eyes. He turns his head and looks up at the birds flying overhead. The lion yawns and stretches up.

Make a pillow with the other hand and fall asleep on the other side. He sleeps there for a minute. He hears something. He opens his eyes and sees a beautiful bird. He stretches his neck turning up to see it, but he is so tired he falls asleep once more.

He opens his eyes and looks up at the moon and stars. He stretches, lies down on the other knee, and falls sound asleep.

#8 The Energy Ball audio script

Energy is all around us in nature and in our bodies. Reach up over your head and take a ball of energy. Bring it down and hold it in front of your chest with your palms facing each other. Close your eyes. Roll the ball. One hand is on top and then the other. Keep your eyes closed and notice the color of the ball. Feel the tingle in your palms.

Now place the ball of energy on top of your head. Stand very tall and straight so it doesn't roll off. Let go. Stay very still. Open your eyes and look at a spot on the earth. Now, carefully balancing the ball on your head, lift one foot a few inches off the ground. Lift it a little bit higher and slowly return it to the earth.

Now lift the other foot. Focus on the root. Lift it a little bit higher. Keep your eyes open, looking at the earth. Concentrate on your roots so you will be steady. Move slowly. Return your foot to the earth.

Bring the ball down from the top of your head and hold it in front of your chest. Close your eyes to stare at the ball again. Let it grow a little bit bigger as you inhale. Separate your arms. Let it grow a bit smaller as you exhale. Bring your hands together. Let it grow bigger again and then smaller.

Now place the energy inside your abdomen. Close your eyes and rest your hands on your abdomen. As you inhale, feel the energy ball grow a bit bigger. Expand your abdomen. As you exhale, let it grow smaller. Feel it move back towards your spine. Inhale. Feel it expand. Exhale. Feel it contract, rolling back towards your spine. Continue to breathe comfortably and feel the gentle wave of energy moving in your body. Your eyes are closed. Nothing is forced.

As you breathe, you focus on the energy. See the color. Sometimes the color changes as you breathe. It might feel warm. Notice how your shoulders begin to relax. They begin to drop down. Feel the muscles of your face relax. Be aware of the energy inside and around you.

Where Did I Feel My Chi Today?

A weekly picture diary is another fun way to experience Tai Chi for Kids. Make copies of the figure below and show where the energy was felt. What did it feel like? What color was it? It might be different every day. The chi is always moving in our body. Is it different when we are feeling tired or happy? In the morning or the evening? It is nice to be aware of our energy shifts. It can help us understand how we feel.

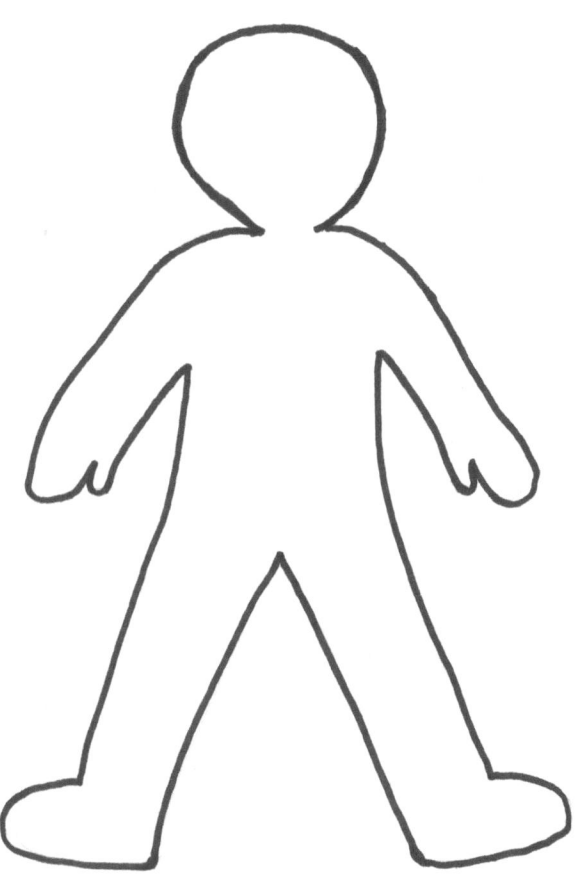

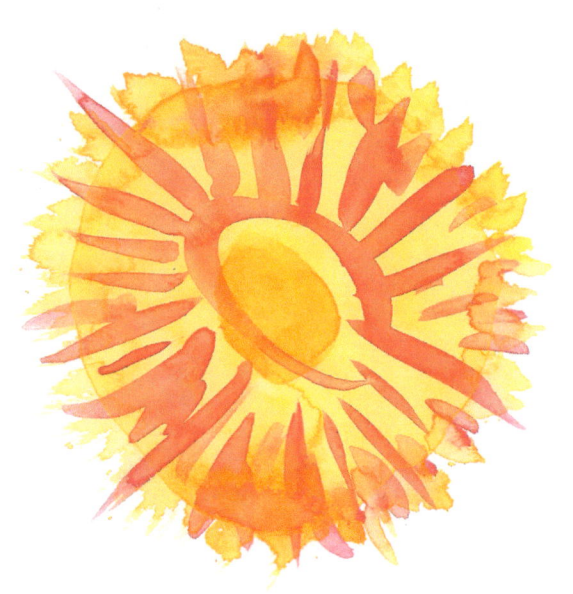

About the Author

Traveling in China in 1991, Cari Shurman accidentally "discovered" the ancient art of Tai Chi. Seeing the graceful movements in parks and classrooms, she was curious. She tried it herself and felt the wonderful flow of *chi* in her body. She realized that Tai Chi could enhance learning, self-esteem, and wellness in her students. After years of study in the US with a variety of teachers, she returned to China twice to deepen her understanding. Then, trying it with her own students, she was very pleased 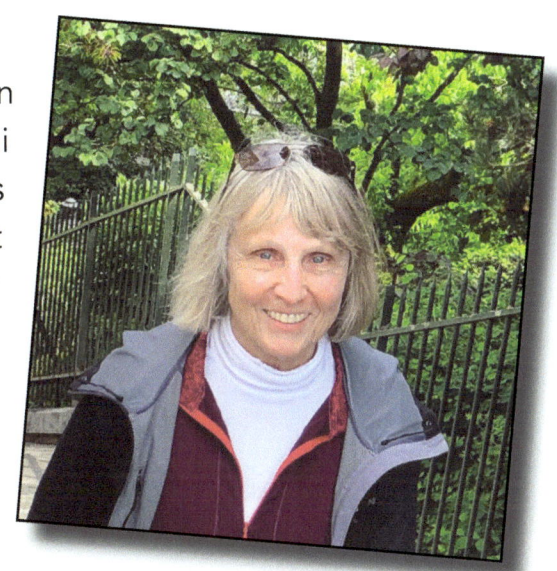 with their reactions and their desire to learn more. This was from both the stressed out high achievers and those with learning challenges who couldn't sit still. The whole class became more focused. She was inspired to develop a program which she called **Tai Chi for Kids©**.

For more than twenty-five years she has been teaching the focus and relaxation of Tai Chi. This book will show you how to bring the wonderful benefits of Tai Chi into your busy lives in just a few minutes a day. It works for all ages.

Shurman has greatly expanded the reach of *Tai Chi for Kids* by training teachers all over the U.S. and in many other countries including Brazil, England, Germany, Canada, South Africa, Myanmar, and Kuwait. Her videos and audio guides make this possible. She worked with teachers in the New York City public schools for twenty-three years. And along the way, she has been on public TV programs and conducted workshops in schools and for other organizations, including the Juvenile Division of the Cape Town Police Department in South Africa.

Shurman says, "What I've learned again and again over decades of teaching is that Tai Chi can change your life!"

www.ingramcontent.com/pod-product-compliance
Lightning Source LLC
Chambersburg PA
CBHW041555120626
46551CB00002B/216